EASY

ANTI-INFLAMMATORY

DIET MEAL-PREP

COOKBOOK

Quick and Tasty Recipes to Boost Your Immune System, Detox Your Body, Reduce Inflammation and Achieve Optimal Health

Brittany Rice

TABLE OF CONTENT

It all began one gloomy winter day when I sat in the doctor's office, receiving yet another prescription for pain medication to alleviate the relentless discomfort that had become my daily companion. I was only in my early 40s, but my body felt twice that age. The diagnosis was chronic inflammation, which had caused a cascade of health issues, from joint pain to fatigue and skin problems. I knew I had to make a change, and that's when I stumbled upon a life-changing solution - an anti-inflammatory diet cookbook.

Deciding to take charge of my life and switch to an anti-inflammatory diet was the first step on my path to better health. I came upon a cookbook that promised to support me all the way; it was full of delectable recipes meant to lower inflammation and enhance general wellbeing. With hope in my heart, I embarked on this transformative journey.

My first experiment was a breakfast recipe called the "Berry Blast Smoothie." This vibrant blend of strawberries, blueberries, and kale was a revelation. As I sipped this green elixir, I couldn't help but be amazed at how something so nutritious could be so delicious. I thought, "Maybe this won't be as tough as I imagined."

I jumped right in and started trying out all the recipes. Every dish, from colorful salads to filling main courses, was a revelation. Everybody in the family started to love the " Ginger and Turmeric Chicken Stir-Fry." The warmth of ginger and the earthy notes of turmeric filled my kitchen, and the satisfying aroma signaled a change not just in my diet but in my life.

Week by week, I noticed subtle changes. My joint pain lessened, my energy levels increased, and my skin began to glow with newfound vitality. The "Roasted Turmeric Almonds" were my go-to snack, providing a delightful crunch while taming inflammation. Each small victory was a testament to the power of this anti-inflammatory diet.

Adopting a new way of eating also brought a fresh perspective on social gatherings. Instead of feeling left out, I started sharing my newfound recipes with friends and family. We discovered that an anti-inflammatory diet wasn't just about health but about embracing the joy of cooking and eating together.

As months passed, I revisited my doctor for a check-up. The results were nothing short of astonishing. My inflammation markers had significantly decreased, and my overall health had improved dramatically. My reliance on pain medications had reduced, and I felt more alive than I had in years. The "Chocolate Avocado Pudding" had become my occasional treat, a reminder of the sweet victories I had achieved.

Today, I am a different person. I no longer feel like a prisoner of chronic inflammation. I am free to pursue my passions and enjoy the simple pleasures of life. I credit this transformation to the anti-inflammatory diet cookbook that introduced me to a world of delicious, healing foods.

In this journey, I discovered that an anti-inflammatory diet wasn't just a change in eating habits; it was a change in my entire lifestyle. The cookbook didn't just provide recipes; it offered a lifeline, a path to renewed vitality. Now, I'm not just eating to live; I'm living to eat - and living life to the fullest.

CHAPTER ONE: BENEFITS OF AN ANTI-INFLAMMATORY DIET

Consuming foods that have been demonstrated to lessen inflammation in the body is the main goal of an anti-inflammatory diet. Although inflammation is a normal reaction to damage or infection, persistent inflammation has been connected to a number of health problems, including chronic illnesses. Among the main advantages of switching to an anti-inflammatory diet are the following:

1. Diminished Probability of Chronic Illnesses: Prolonged inflammation is frequently the root cause of numerous chronic ailments, such as diabetes, cancer, heart disease, and autoimmune disorders. Reduced risk of developing these conditions can be achieved by following an anti-inflammatory diet.

2. Joint Pain Relief: Inflammation can cause joint pain and stiffness, such as in the case of arthritis. An anti-inflammatory diet can help reduce joint inflammation, alleviate pain, and improve mobility.

3. Weight Management: Obesity is associated with increased inflammation in the body. An anti-inflammatory diet can aid in weight management by promoting healthier food choices and reducing the risk of overeating.

4. Better Digestive Health: Prolonged inflammation can make inflammatory bowel conditions like Crohn's disease and ulcerative colitis worse. Foods high in antioxidants can help calm the digestive tract and lessen discomfort.

5. Increased Heart Health: Heart disease is exacerbated by chronic inflammation. A diet high in anti-inflammatory foods can help lower blood pressure, cholesterol, and enhance heart health in general.

6. Enhanced Brain Health: Some research suggests that chronic inflammation may play a role in cognitive decline and neurodegenerative diseases like Alzheimer's.

An anti-inflammatory diet rich in antioxidants and omega-3 fatty acids can support brain health.

7. Skin Health: Irritation can make skin disorders worse, such as eczema, psoriasis, and acne. Eating foods high in anti-inflammatory compounds can help to improve skin health and appearance.

8. Balanced Blood Sugar: An anti-inflammatory diet can help regulate blood sugar levels, reducing the risk of insulin resistance and type 2 diabetes.

9. Increased Energy and Vitality: Many people report feeling more energetic and vital when following an anti-inflammatory diet. It can reduce fatigue and promote a sense of well-being.

10. Long-Term Health and Well-Being: By reducing inflammation in the body, an anti-inflammatory diet can contribute to overall long-term health and well-being, potentially increasing lifespan and quality of life.

An anti-inflammatory diet typically includes foods rich in antioxidants, such as fruits and vegetables, as well as foods containing healthy fats like omega-3 fatty acids found in fatty fish. It also emphasizes whole grains, lean proteins, and limits or eliminates processed foods, sugar, and unhealthy fats. It's important to note that while an anti-inflammatory diet can offer numerous health benefits, it is not a replacement for medical treatment when needed. Individuals with specific health concerns should consult with a healthcare professional before making significant dietary changes.

THE BASICS OF AN ANTI-INFLAMMATORY DIET

Anti-Inflammatory Foods: An anti-inflammatory diet is primarily composed of foods that are known to have anti-inflammatory properties. These foods typically include:

- Fruits and Vegetables: Particularly those rich in antioxidants like vitamin C, vitamin E, and beta-carotene. Leafy greens, berries, and vibrant vegetables are all great options.

- Fatty Fish: Fish such as salmon, mackerel, and sardines are high in omega-3 fatty acids, which have potent anti-inflammatory effects.

- Nuts and Seeds: Almonds, walnuts, flaxseeds, and chia seeds provide healthy fats and antioxidants that combat inflammation.

- Whole Grains: Foods like brown rice, quinoa, and whole wheat contain fiber and phytonutrients that reduce inflammation.

- Healthy Fats: Olive oil, avocados, and nuts contain monounsaturated fats and are known for their anti-inflammatory properties.

- Spices and Herbs: Turmeric, ginger, garlic, and green tea are often incorporated into an anti-inflammatory diet due to their anti-inflammatory and antioxidant compounds.

Foods to Limit or Avoid:

Equally important in an anti-inflammatory diet is the avoidance or limitation of foods that can promote inflammation. These typically include:

- Processed Foods: Highly processed foods often contain trans fats, excessive sugar, and refined carbohydrates, all of which can contribute to inflammation.

- Sugary Beverages: Sodas and sugary drinks are associated with inflammation and should be minimized.

- Red and Processed Meats: High consumption of red and processed meats has been linked to inflammation and chronic diseases.

- Excessive Saturated Fats: Limit foods high in saturated fats, such as fatty cuts of meat, full-fat dairy products, and some tropical oils.

Be Mindful of Dairy and Gluten:

- Some individuals may be sensitive to dairy and gluten, which can contribute to inflammation. Experiment with dairy alternatives and gluten-free options if you suspect they might be problematic for you.

Stay Hydrated:

- Drinking enough water is essential for good health. Drinking water helps flush toxins and promotes a balanced inflammatory response.

Moderation is Key: - While these dietary guidelines are beneficial, moderation is essential. Enjoying a balanced and varied diet is crucial for long-term success and satisfaction.

Balanced Eating:

An anti-inflammatory diet emphasizes a balanced and varied intake of these anti-inflammatory foods. Meals should be rich in vegetables, include a moderate amount of fruits and whole grains, and incorporate lean protein sources, such as poultry and plant-based proteins like legumes and tofu.

Hydration:

Staying well-hydrated is a fundamental aspect of an anti-inflammatory diet. Drinking water and herbal teas can help flush toxins from the body and support overall health.

Lifestyle Factors:

In addition to dietary changes, other lifestyle factors like regular physical activity, stress management, and adequate sleep play crucial roles in reducing inflammation and maintaining a healthy body.

BUILDING A BALANCED PLATE

Creating a balanced plate is a fundamental principle of healthy eating. It ensures that you provide your body with a wide range of essential nutrients, maintain energy levels, and promote overall well-being. Whether you're following a specific dietary plan or simply aiming for a healthier lifestyle, understanding how to build a balanced plate is key. Here are some essential guidelines to help you achieve this:

1. Include a Variety of Food Groups:

   - Your plate should represent a diversity of food groups to ensure you receive a broad spectrum of nutrients. This typically includes vegetables, fruits, lean proteins, whole grains, and healthy fats.

2. Vegetables Take Center Stage:

   - Vegetables should cover a significant portion of your plate. They are rich in vitamins, minerals, and dietary fiber while being low in calories. Aim for a colorful array of vegetables to maximize the variety of nutrients you consume.

3. Add Lean Proteins:

   - Lean protein sources, such as poultry, fish, tofu, legumes, and lean cuts of meat, contribute to muscle health and satiety. Additionally, they include vital amino acids that are required for a number of body processes.

4. Incorporate Whole Grains:

   - Whole grains like brown rice, quinoa, oats, and whole wheat pasta provide complex carbohydrates, fiber, and essential nutrients. They help regulate blood sugar and maintain energy levels.

5. Healthy Fats in Moderation:

   - Incorporate healthy fats like avocados, olive oil, nuts, and seeds in moderation. These fats are vital for brain health and the absorption of fat-soluble vitamins (A, D, E, and K).

6. Portion Control: Pay attention to serving sizes to avoid consuming too much food. Using smaller plates can help

you control portion sizes while making your plate appear full and satisfying.

7. Balance Macros:

   - Ensure a balance between macronutrients, including carbohydrates, proteins, and fats. The exact ratio may vary depending on your individual needs and dietary preferences.

8. Hydrate with Water:

   - Don't forget to hydrate. Water is necessary for healthy digestion, metabolism, and general wellbeing. Limiting sugar-filled beverages and excessive caffeine is also a smart idea.

9. Listen to Your Body:

   - Observe your body's signals of hunger and fullness. You can make healthier food choices and prevent overeating by eating with awareness and intuition.

10. Personalize to Your Needs: Your plate should be customized to meet your specific needs, accounting for

things like age, degree of activity, and dietary restrictions. Consult with a registered dietitian for personalized guidance if needed.

Building a balanced plate is not about strict rules but about making choices that support your health and well-being. It's a flexible and sustainable approach to eating that can be adapted to various dietary preferences and lifestyles. Remember that achieving balance is a dynamic process, and what works best for you may change over time. By focusing on nutrient-dense foods and mindful eating, you can enjoy a satisfying and nourishing meal while promoting your long-term health.

CHAPTER 2: BREAKFAST DELIGHTS

1. Berry Blast Smoothie

Prep and Cooking Time: 5 minutes

Nutritional Information (approximate):

- Calories: 250

- Protein: 15g

- Carbohydrates: 30g

- Fiber: 9g

- Fat: 8g

Ingredients:

- 1 cup mixed berries (strawberries, blueberries, raspberries)
- 1/2 cup spinach or kale
- 1/2 cup plain Greek yogurt
- 1 tablespoon chia seeds
- 1/2 cup almond milk
- 1/2 teaspoon turmeric
- Honey (optional, for sweetness)

Instructions:

1. Combine all ingredients in a blender.

2. Blend until smooth and creamy.

3. Adjust sweetness with honey if desired.

2. Avocado and Tomato Breakfast Toast

Prep and Cooking Time: 10 minutes

Nutritional Information (Approximate):

- Calories: 330

- Protein: 6g

- Carbohydrates: 25g

- Fiber: 8g

- Fat: 23g

Ingredients:

- 2 slices of whole-grain bread

- 1 ripe avocado

- 1 small tomato, sliced

- 1 tablespoon olive oil

- Salt and pepper to taste

- A sprinkle of red pepper flakes (optional)

Instructions:

1. Toast the bread until golden brown.

2. After mashing the avocado, evenly distribute it over the toast.

3. Top with tomato slices.

4. Drizzle with olive oil and season with salt, pepper, and red pepper flakes if desired.

3. Quinoa Breakfast Bowl

Prep and Cooking Time: 15 minutes (if quinoa is pre-cooked)

Nutritional Information (Approximate):

- Calories: 350

- Protein: 10g

- Carbohydrates: 45g

- Fiber: 6g

- Fat: 15g

Ingredients:

- 1/2 cup cooked quinoa

- 1/2 cup mixed berries (e.g., blueberries, strawberries)

- 1/4 cup chopped nuts (e.g., almonds, walnuts)

- 1 tablespoon honey or maple syrup

- 1/4 cup plain Greek yogurt

- 1/2 teaspoon ground cinnamon

Instructions:

1. Cook quinoa according to package instructions.

2. In a bowl, layer the cooked quinoa, mixed berries, and chopped nuts.

3. Drizzle with honey or maple syrup, and top with Greek yogurt.

4. Sprinkle it with ground cinnamon.

4. Turmeric and Ginger Oatmeal

Prep and Cooking Time: 10 minutes

Nutritional Information (approximate):

- Calories: 280

- Protein: 6g

- Carbohydrates: 51g

- Fiber: 7g

- Fat: 6g

Ingredients:

- 1/2 cup rolled oats

- 1 cup almond milk

- 1/2 teaspoon ground turmeric

- 1/2 teaspoon grated ginger

- 1/4 teaspoon cinnamon

- 1/4 cup chopped dried apricots

- 1 tablespoon honey (optional)

Instructions:

1. In a saucepan, combine oats, almond milk, turmeric, ginger, and cinnamon.

2. Cook over medium heat, stirring occasionally, until the oats are creamy and cooked to your liking.

3. Top with dried apricots and honey, if desired.

5. Chia Seed Pudding

Prep and Cooking Time: 5 minutes (plus chilling time)

Nutritional Information (Approximate):

- Calories: 230

- Protein: 6g

- Carbohydrates: 31g

- Fiber: 13g

- Fat: 9g

Ingredients:

- 3 tablespoons chia seeds

- 1 cup almond milk

- 1/2 teaspoon vanilla extract

- 1/2 cup mixed berries

- 1 tablespoon honey (optional)

Instructions:

1. In a jar or bowl, combine chia seeds, almond milk, and vanilla ,Extract.

2. Stir well and refrigerate overnight (or at least for 4 hours) to allow the chia seeds to absorb the liquid and thicken.

3. In the morning, top with mixed berries and honey if desired.

6. Mediterranean Breakfast Bowl

Prep and Cooking Time: 15 minutes (if quinoa is pre-cooked)

Nutritional Information (Approximate):

- Calories: 350

- Protein: 10g

- Carbohydrates: 30g

- Fiber: 4g

- Fat: 20g

Ingredients:

- 1/2 cup cooked quinoa

- 1/4 cup diced cucumber

- 1/4 cup diced tomatoes

- 2 tablespoons diced red onion

- 2 tablespoons crumbled feta cheese

- Kalamata olives, pitted and sliced (to taste)

- Fresh parsley, chopped

- 1 tablespoon extra-virgin olive oil

- Lemon juice to taste

- Salt and pepper to taste

Instructions:

1. In a bowl, combine quinoa, cucumber, tomatoes, red onion, and feta cheese.

2. Top with olives and fresh parsley.

3. Drizzle with extra-virgin olive oil, lemon juice, and season with salt and pepper.

7. Spinach and Mushroom Omelette

Prep and Cooking Time: 15 minutes

Nutritional Information (Approximate):

- Calories: 280

- Protein: 21g

- Carbohydrates: 9g

- Fiber: 2g

- Fat: 19g

Ingredients:

- 2 large eggs

- 1 cup fresh spinach

- 1/2 cup sliced mushrooms

- 1/4 cup diced bell peppers

- 1/4 cup diced onions

- 1/4 cup shredded low-fat mozzarella cheese

- Salt and pepper to taste

- Olive oil for cooking

Instructions:

1. In a bowl, beat the eggs and season with salt and pepper.

2. A little bit of olive oil has been added to a non-stick skillet that has been heated over medium heat.

3. Sauté the mushrooms, bell peppers, and onions until they soften.

4. Add the fresh spinach to the skillet and cook until wilted.

5. Pour the beaten eggs over the vegetables and cook until set.

6. Sprinkle it with mozzarella cheese and fold the omelet in half.

8. Smashed Avo and Poached Eggs on Whole-Grain Toast

Prep and Cooking Time: 15 minutes

Nutritional Information (Approximate):

- Calories: 350

- Protein: 13g

- Carbohydrates: 29g

- Fiber: 9g

- Fat: 22g

Ingredients:

- 2 slices of whole-grain toast

- 1 ripe avocado

- 2 poached eggs

- Salt and pepper to taste

- A sprinkle of red pepper flakes (optional)

Instructions:

1. Golden brown toast the whole-grain bread.

2. After mashing the avocado, evenly distribute it over the toast.

3. Top each slice with a poached egg.

4. Season with salt, pepper, and red pepper flakes if desired.

9. Blueberry Almond Chia Pudding

Prep and Cooking Time: 5 minutes (plus chilling time)

Nutritional Information (Approximate):

- Calories: 250

- Protein: 6g

- Carbohydrates: 29g

- Fiber: 10g

- Fat: 14g

Ingredients:

- 3 tablespoons chia seeds

- 1 cup almond milk

- 1/2 teaspoon almond extract

- 1/4 cup fresh blueberries

- 1 tablespoon sliced almonds

- 1 tablespoon honey (optional)

Instructions:

1. In a jar or bowl, combine chia seeds, almond milk, and almond extract.

2. Stir well and refrigerate overnight (or at least for 4 hours) to allow the chia seeds to absorb the liquid and thicken.

3. In the morning, top with fresh blueberries, sliced almonds, and honey if desired.

10. Veggie Breakfast Burrito

Prep and Cooking Time:20 minutes

Nutritional Information (Approximate):

- Calories: 390

- Protein: 22g

- Carbohydrates: 40g

- Fiber: 10g

- Fat: 15g

Ingredients:

- 2 large whole-grain tortillas

- 4 large eggs, beaten

- 1/2 cup diced bell peppers

- 1/4 cup diced red onion

- 1/2 cup black beans, drained and rinsed

- 1/4 cup salsa

- 1/4 cup shredded low-fat cheddar cheese

- Salt and pepper to taste

- Olive oil for cooking

Instructions:

1. Heat a non-stick skillet over medium heat and add a small amount of olive oil.

2. Sauté the diced bell peppers and red onion until they soften.

3. Include the whisked eggs and cook through by scrambling.

4. Warm the whole-grain tortillas in a dry skillet or microwave.

5. Assemble the burritos by layering the scrambled eggs, black beans, salsa, and cheddar cheese.

6. Fold the sides and roll up the tortilla to create a burrito.

CHAPTER 3: SATISFYING SALADS & SOUPS

1. Kale and Blueberry Salad

Prep and Cooking Time: 20 minutes

Nutritional Info (per serving):

- Calories: 300

- Protein: 6g

- Carbohydrates: 25g

- Fat: 21g

- Fiber: 4g

Ingredients:

- 4 cups chopped kale

- 1 cup fresh blueberries

- 1/2 cup chopped walnuts

- 1/4 cup crumbled feta cheese

- 2 tablespoons extra-virgin olive oil

- 2 tablespoons balsamic vinegar

- 1 teaspoon honey (optional)

- Salt and pepper to taste

Instructions:

1. Chopped kale, blueberries, walnuts, and feta cheese should all be combined in a large salad bowl.

2. Olive oil, balsamic vinegar, honey (if using), salt, and pepper should all be combined in a small bowl.

Pour the dressing over the salad and mix everything together.ng.

4. Let the salad sit for about 15 minutes to allow the flavors to meld.

5. Serve and enjoy!

2. Tomato Basil Soup

Prep and Cooking Time: 45 minutes

Nutritional Info (per serving):

- Calories: 120

- Protein: 2g

- Carbohydrates: 14g

- Fat: 7g

- Fiber: 3g

Ingredients:

- 6 ripe tomatoes, chopped

- 1 onion, diced

- 3 cloves garlic, minced

- 1/4 cup fresh basil leaves, chopped

- 2 cups vegetable broth

- 2 tablespoons olive oil

- Salt and pepper to taste

Instructions:

1. Warm up the olive oil in a big pot on medium heat. Saute the garlic and onions until they become tender.

2. After adding the chopped tomatoes, cook for about ten minutes, or until they begin to break down.

3. Once the vegetable broth has been added, bring the mixture to a boil. For twenty to twenty-five minutes, simmer, covered, over low heat.

4. Smoothly puree the soup using an immersion blender or a standard blender.

5. Add the fresh basil and add some salt and pepper to taste.

6. Serve hot and garnish with extra basil leaves.

3. Mediterranean Quinoa Salad

Prep and Cooking Time: 30 minutes

Nutritional Info (per serving):

- Calories: 350

- Protein: 8g

- Carbohydrates: 28g

- Fat: 24g

- Fiber: 4g

Ingredients:

- 1 cup cooked quinoa

- 1 cup cherry tomatoes, halved

- 1 cucumber, diced

- 1/2 cup of pitted and sliced Kalamata olives

- 1/4 cup red onion, finely chopped

- 1/4 cup crumbled feta cheese

- 2 tablespoons extra-virgin olive oil

- 2 tablespoons lemon juice

- 1 teaspoon dried oregano

- Salt and pepper to taste

Instructions:

1. In a large bowl, combine cooked quinoa, cherry tomatoes, cucumber, olives, red onion, and feta cheese.

2. In a small bowl, whisk together olive oil, lemon juice, dried oregano, salt, and pepper.

Pour the dressing over the salad and mix everything together.ng.

4. Chill the salad for at least 30 minutes before serving.

4. Turmeric and Ginger Oatmeal Soup

Prep and Cooking Time: 30 minutes

Nutritional Info (per serving):

- Calories: 200

- Protein: 6g

- Carbohydrates: 38g

- Fat: 3g

- Fiber: 6g

Ingredients:

- 1 cup rolled oats

- 4 cups vegetable broth

- 1 tablespoon turmeric

- 1 tablespoon grated fresh ginger

- 1/2 cup diced carrots

- 1/2 cup diced celery

- Salt and pepper to taste

- Chopped fresh cilantro for garnish (optional)

Instructions:

1. In a large pot, combine rolled oats, vegetable broth, turmeric, grated ginger, diced carrots, and celery.

2. Bring the mixture to a boil, then reduce the heat and simmer for 15-20 minutes, or until the oats and vegetables are tender.

3. Season with salt and pepper to taste.

4. Serve hot, garnished with fresh cilantro if desired.

5. Butternut Squash and Red Lentil Soup

Prep and Cooking Time: 45 minutes

Nutritional Info (per serving):

- Calories: 250

- Protein: 10g

- Carbohydrates: 48g

- Fat: 4g

- Fiber: 9g

Ingredients:

- 1 butternut squash, peeled and cubed

- 1 cup red lentils

- 1 onion, diced

- 2 cloves garlic, minced

- 1 teaspoon ground cumin

- 1 teaspoon ground coriander

- 6 cups vegetable broth

- 2 tablespoons olive oil

- Salt and pepper to taste

Instructions:

1. In a large pot, heat olive oil over medium heat. Add diced onions and garlic and sauté until soft.

2. Incorporate chopped butternut squash, red lentils, ground coriander, and ground cumin. Stir for several minutes.

3. After adding the vegetable broth, heat the mixture until it boils. Once the butternut squash and lentils are soft, reduce the heat, cover, and simmer for 25 to 30 minutes.

4. Puree the soup until it is smooth using an immersion blender or a standard blender.

5. To taste, add salt and pepper for seasoning.

6. Present warm.

6. Beet and Spinach Salad

Prep and Cooking Time: 40 minutes (includes roasting the beets)

Nutritional Info (per serving):

- Calories: 280

- Protein: 6g

- Carbohydrates: 15g

- Fat: 21g

- Fiber: 4g

Ingredients:

- 2 cups baby spinach leaves

- 1 medium beet, roasted and cubed

- 1/4 cup crumbled goat cheese

- 1/4 cup chopped walnuts

- 2 tablespoons extra-virgin olive oil

- 1 tablespoon balsamic vinegar

- 1 teaspoon honey (optional)

- Salt and pepper to taste

Instructions:

1. In a large salad bowl, combine baby spinach, roasted beets, goat cheese, and chopped walnuts.

2. In a small bowl, whisk together olive oil, balsamic vinegar, honey (if using), salt, and pepper.

3. Shake to mix the salad after adding the dressing.

4. Serve and enjoy!

7. Anti-Inflammatory Turmeric Soup

Prep and Cooking Time: 40 minutes

Nutritional Info (per serving):

- Calories: 280

- Protein: 3g

- Carbohydrates: 18g

- Fat: 23g

- Fiber: 5g

Ingredients:

- 1 tablespoon coconut oil

- 1 onion, chopped

- 2 cloves garlic, minced

- 1 teaspoon ground turmeric

- 1 teaspoon ground ginger

- 3 carrots, diced

- 3 cups vegetable broth

- 1 can (15 oz) coconut milk

- Salt and pepper to taste

- Fresh cilantro for garnish (optional)

Instructions:

1. In a large pot, the coconut oil should be heated over medium heat. Saute the chopped garlic and onions until they become tender.

2. Incorporate chopped carrots, ground ginger, and turmeric. Stir for a couple of minutes.

3. Add the vegetable broth and heat the mixture until it reaches a boiling point. After lowering the heat and covering the carrots, simmer them for twenty to twenty-five minutes, or until they become soft.

4. Use a regular blender or an immersion blender to puree the soup smoothly.

5. Add the coconut milk to the soup and heat it through without boiling it. To taste, add salt and pepper for seasoning.

6. Garnish with fresh cilantro if desired.

8. Cucumber and Mint Tzatziki Salad

Prep and Cooking Time: 15 minutes

Nutritional Info (per serving):

- Calories: 120

- Protein: 6g

- Carbohydrates: 10g

- Fat: 7g

- Fiber: 1g

Ingredients:

- 2 cucumbers, peeled, seeded, and diced

- 1 cup plain Greek yogurt

- 2 tablespoons fresh mint, chopped

- 1 clove garlic, minced

- 1 tablespoon lemon juice

- 1 tablespoon extra-virgin olive oil

- Salt and pepper to taste

Instructions:

1. In a bowl, combine diced cucumbers, plain Greek yogurt, chopped mint, minced garlic, lemon juice, and olive oil.

2. Stir to combine all the ingredients.

3. Season with salt and pepper to taste.

4. Chill the tzatziki salad for at least 30 minutes before serving.

9. Lentil and Sweet Potato Salad

Prep and Cooking Time: 45 minutes (includes roasting the sweet potatoes)

Nutritional Info (per serving):

- Calories: 300

- Protein: 8g

- Carbohydrates: 45g

- Fat: 10g

- Fiber: 10g

Ingredients:

- 1 cup cooked green or brown lentils

- 2 cups roasted sweet potatoes, cubed

- 1 red bell pepper, diced

- 1/4 cup red onion, finely chopped

- 2 tablespoons extra-virgin olive oil

- 2 tablespoons balsamic vinegar

- 1 teaspoon Dijon mustard

- Salt and pepper to taste

Instructions:

1. In a large salad bowl, combine cooked lentils, roasted sweet potatoes, red bell pepper, and red onion.

2. In a small bowl, whisk together olive oil, balsamic vinegar, Dijon mustard, salt, and pepper.

Pour the dressing over the salad and mix everything together.

4. Serve and enjoy!

10. Golden Milk Soup

Prep and Cooking Time: 40 minutes

Nutritional Info (per serving):

- Calories: 250

- Protein: 3g

- Carbohydrates: 18g

- Fat: 23g

- Fiber: 5g

Ingredients:

- 1 tablespoon coconut oil

- 1 onion, chopped

- 2 cloves garlic, minced

- 1 teaspoon ground turmeric

- 1 teaspoon ground ginger

- 4 cups vegetable broth

- 1 can (15 oz) coconut milk

- Salt and pepper to taste

- Fresh cilantro for garnish (optional)

Instructions:

1. In a large pot, heat coconut oil over medium heat. Saute the chopped garlic and onions until they become tender.

2. Grind in the ginger and turmeric. For a few minutes, stir.

3. After adding the vegetable broth, raise the temperature to a boil. For twenty to twenty-five minutes, simmer, covered, on low heat.

4. Puree the soup until it is smooth using an immersion blender or a standard blender.

5. Stir in the coconut milk and warm the soup without boiling. Season with salt and pepper to taste.

6. Garnish with fresh cilantro if desired.

CHAPTER 4: WHOLESOME MAIN COURSES

1. Baked Salmon with Lemon and Dill

Prep and Cooking Time: About 30 minutes

Nutritional Info (per serving):

- Calories: 330

- Protein: 35g

- Fat: 19g

- Carbohydrates: 4g

- Fiber: 1g

Ingredients:

- 4 salmon filets (6-8 oz each)

- 2 lemons, sliced

- 2 tablespoons fresh dill, chopped

- 2 cloves garlic, minced

- 2 tablespoons olive oil

- Salt and pepper to taste

Instructions:

1. Turn the oven's temperature up to 375°F (190°C).

2. Every salmon filet should be placed on a piece of aluminum foil. Add pepper and salt for seasoning.

3. Combine the dill, olive oil, and minced garlic in a small bowl. Drizzle this mixture over the salmon.

4. Place a slice of lemon over each filet.

5. Wrap the foil around the salmon to create a packet.

6. Bake for 15-20 minutes, or until the salmon flakes easily with a fork.

2. Turmeric and Ginger Chicken Stir-Fry

Prep and Cooking Time: About 30 minutes

Nutritional Info (per serving):

- Calories: 330

- Protein: 30g

- Fat: 12g

- Carbohydrates: 18g

- Fiber: 4g

Ingredients:

- 2 boneless, skinless chicken breasts, sliced

- 2 tablespoons olive oil

- 1 onion, sliced

- 1 red bell pepper, sliced

- 1 zucchini, sliced

- 1 tablespoon fresh ginger, minced

- 1 tablespoon turmeric powder

- 2 tablespoons low-sodium soy sauce

- Salt and pepper to taste

Instructions:

1. On medium-high heat, warm the olive oil in a big pan or wok.

2. Cook the chicken until browned after adding it. Take out and place aside.

3. Add the bell pepper, onion, and zucchini to the same pan. Stir-fry for tenderness.

4. Return the cooked chicken to the pan with the ginger, turmeric, and soy sauce.

5. Cook, stirring frequently, for a further two to three minutes.

3. Lentil and Sweet Potato Curry

Prep and Cooking Time: About 45 minutes

Nutritional Info (per serving):

- Calories: 380

- Protein: 14g

- Fat: 16g

- Carbohydrates: 50g

- Fiber: 10g

Ingredients:

- A cup of dried lentils, either brown or green

- 2 sweet potatoes, peeled and diced

- 1 onion, chopped

- 2 cloves garlic, minced

- 2 tablespoons curry powder

- 1 can (14 oz) of diced tomatoes

- 1 can (14 oz) of coconut milk

- 2 tablespoons olive oil

- Salt and pepper to taste

Instructions:

1. In a large pot, heat the olive oil and sauté the onions and garlic until softened.

2. Add the curry powder and cook for a minute until fragrant.

3. Stir in the lentils, sweet potatoes, diced tomatoes, and coconut milk. Add salt and pepper.

4. Simmer for 25-30 minutes, or until lentils and sweet potatoes are tender.

4. Quinoa and Chickpea Stuffed Bell Peppers

Prep and Cooking Time: About 45 minutes

Nutritional Info (per serving):

- Calories: 350

- Protein: 12g

- Fat: 2g

- Carbohydrates: 72g

- Fiber: 12g

Ingredients:

- 4 bell peppers

- 1 cup quinoa, cooked

- 1 can (15 oz) of chickpeas, drained and rinsed

- 1 cup diced tomatoes

- 1/2 cup fresh spinach, chopped

- 2 cloves garlic, minced

- 1 teaspoon cumin

- Salt and pepper to taste

Instructions:

1. Preheat the oven to 375°F (190°C).

2. Slice the bell peppers in half, then take out the seeds and membranes.

3. In a bowl, mix cooked quinoa, chickpeas, diced tomatoes, spinach, garlic, and cumin. Add salt and pepper.

4. Stuff each bell pepper with the quinoa and chickpea mixture.

5. Place stuffed peppers in a baking dish, cover with foil, and bake for 25-30 minutes.

5. Mediterranean Quinoa Salad

Prep and Cooking Time: About 20 minutes

Nutritional Info (per serving):

- Calories: 350

- Protein: 9g

- Fat: 18g

- Carbohydrates: 39g

- Fiber: 6g

Ingredients:

- 1 cup quinoa, cooked

- 1 cucumber, diced

- 1 cup cherry tomatoes, halved

- 1/2 red onion, finely chopped

- 1/2 cup Kalamata olives, pitted and sliced

- 1/4 cup fresh parsley, chopped

- 1/4 cup feta cheese, crumbled

- 3 tablespoons olive oil

- 2 tablespoons lemon juice

- Salt and pepper to taste

Instructions:

1. Quinoa, cucumbers, cherry tomatoes, red onions, olives, and parsley should all be combined in a big bowl.

2. Lemon juice and olive oil should be combined in a small bowl. Drizzle this over the salad.

3. Include the feta cheese crumbles and mix them in gently.

4. Season with salt and pepper to taste.

6. Grilled Chicken and Vegetable Skewers

Prep and Cooking Time: About 30 minutes

Nutritional Info (per serving):

- Calories: 280

- Protein: 28g

- Fat: 11g

- Carbohydrates: 18g

- Fiber: 4g

Ingredients:

- 2 chicken breasts, sliced into cubes, without the bones and skin

- Chopped bell peppers, zucchini, and red onions

- 2 tablespoons olive oil

- 1 teaspoon dried oregano

- 1 teaspoon garlic powder

- Salt and pepper to taste

Instructions:

1. In a bowl, mix the olive oil, oregano, garlic powder, salt, and pepper.

2. Thread the chicken and vegetable pieces onto skewers.

3. Brush the skewers with the olive oil mixture.

4. Grill the skewers over medium heat for about 10-15 minutes, turning occasionally, until the chicken is cooked through and the vegetables are tender.

7. Spinach and Chickpea Stuffed Sweet Potatoes

Prep and Cooking Time: About 1 hour

Nutritional Info (per serving):

- Calories: 330

- Protein: 10g

- Fat: 9g

- Carbohydrates: 53g

- Fiber: 10g

Ingredients:

- 4 medium sweet potatoes

- 1 can (15 oz) of chickpeas, drained and rinsed

- 2 cups fresh spinach

- 1/4 cup feta cheese, crumbled

- 2 tablespoons olive oil

- 1 teaspoon cumin

- Salt and pepper to taste

Instructions:

1. Preheat the oven to 400°F (200°C).

2. Prick the sweet potatoes with a fork and bake for 45-60 minutes or until they are tender.

3. While the sweet potatoes are baking, heat olive oil in a pan. Add spinach and sauté until wilted.

4. In a bowl, combine chickpeas, sautéed spinach, feta cheese, cumin, salt, and pepper.

5. Once the sweet potatoes are done, slice them open and stuff with the chickpea and spinach mixture.

8. Quinoa and Black Bean Bowl with Avocado

Prep and Cooking Time: About 20 minutes

Nutritional Info (per serving):

- Calories: 390

- Protein: 13g

- Fat: 13g

- Carbohydrates: 59g

- Fiber: 13g

Ingredients:

- 1 cup quinoa, cooked

- 1 can (15 oz) of rinsed and drained black beans

- 1 avocado, sliced

- 1 cup cherry tomatoes, halved

- 1/2 cup corn kernels (fresh, frozen, or canned)

- 1/4 cup fresh cilantro, chopped

- 2 tablespoons lime juice

- Salt and pepper to taste

Instructions:

1. In a bowl, combine cooked quinoa, black beans, avocado, cherry tomatoes, and corn.

2. In a small bowl, whisk together lime juice, salt, and pepper.

3. Drizzle the lime dressing over the quinoa and black bean mixture.

4. Top with fresh cilantro.

9. Baked Turmeric and Ginger Tofu with Broccoli

Prep and Cooking Time: About 40 minutes

Nutritional Info (per serving):

- Calories: 330

- Protein: 16g

- Fat: 22g

- Carbohydrates: 19g

- Fiber: 5g

Ingredients:

- 1 block of extra-firm tofu, cubed

- 2 cups broccoli florets

- 2 tablespoons olive oil

- 1 teaspoon turmeric powder

- 1 teaspoon fresh ginger, minced

- Salt and pepper to taste

Instructions:

1. Preheat the oven to 375°F (190°C).

2. In a bowl, mix olive oil, turmeric, ginger, salt, and pepper.

3. Toss the tofu cubes and broccoli in the olive oil mixture.

4. Spread the tofu and broccoli on a baking sheet and bake for 20-25 minutes, or until the tofu is golden and the broccoli is tender.

10. Stuffed Portobello Mushrooms with Quinoa and Spinach

Prep and Cooking Time: About 45 minutes

Nutritional Info (per serving):

- Calories: 280

- Protein: 12g

- Fat: 10g

- Carbohydrates: 38g

- Fiber: 6g

Ingredients:

- 4 large portobello mushrooms

- 1 cup quinoa, cooked

- 2 cups fresh spinach

- 1/2 cup grated Parmesan cheese

- 2 cloves garlic, minced

- 2 tablespoons olive oil

- Salt and pepper to taste

Instructions:

Set the oven's temperature to 375°F, or 190°C.

2. Remove the stems and gills from the portobello mushrooms.

3. In a pan, heat olive oil and sauté the garlic and spinach until wilted.

4. Grated Parmesan cheese, sautéed spinach, and cooked quinoa should all be combined in a bowl. Include pepper and salt.

5. Ladle the quinoa mixture into the portobello mushrooms.

6. The mushrooms should bake for 20 to 25 minutes after being placed on a baking sheet.

CHAPTER 5: MEAL PLANS & TIPS

Adopting an anti-inflammatory diet can have numerous health benefits, but it requires thoughtful meal planning and a few practical strategies. Here are some meal planning and tips to help you successfully follow an anti-inflammatory diet:

1. Embrace Variety:

   - Incorporate a diverse range of fruits, vegetables, whole grains, lean proteins, and healthy fats into your meals. Different foods provide different anti-inflammatory nutrients.

2. Prioritize Fruits and Vegetables:

   - Make vegetables and fruits the star of your plate. They are rich in antioxidants and phytonutrients that combat inflammation. Aim for at least five servings a day.

3. Choose the Right Fats:

- Opt for sources of healthy fats, such as avocados, olive oil, nuts, and fatty fish. These fats contain omega-3 fatty acids and monounsaturated fats, which have anti-inflammatory properties.

4. Include Omega-3 Rich Foods:

   - Fatty fish like salmon, mackerel, and trout are excellent sources of omega-3s. Consider having fish at least twice a week. If you don't eat fish, incorporate flax seeds, chia seeds, and walnuts into your diet.

5. Whole Grains Over Refined Grains:

   - Replace refined grains with whole grains like brown rice, quinoa, oats, and whole wheat pasta. These provide fiber and essential nutrients that help regulate blood sugar and reduce inflammation.

6. Lean Protein Sources:

   - Opt for lean proteins like skinless poultry, tofu, and legumes. These sources are lower in saturated fat and can be excellent additions to anti-inflammatory meals.

7. Limit Sugar and Processed Foods:

   - Reduce or eliminate added sugars and processed foods from your diet. These can trigger inflammation. Read food labels and be mindful of hidden sugars.

8. Spice It Up:

   - Include anti-inflammatory spices like turmeric, ginger, and cinnamon in your cooking. These spices can add flavor and health benefits to your meals.

9. Practice Portion Control:

   - Pay attention to portion sizes to avoid overeating. Use smaller plates to help control portion sizes while making your plate appear full and satisfying.

10. Plan Your Meals:

   - Plan your meals and snacks ahead of time to ensure you have nutritious options readily available. This reduces the temptation to reach for unhealthy choices when you're hungry.

11. Hydrate with Water:

- Drink plenty of water throughout the day. Proper hydration is essential for digestion, metabolism, and overall health. It can help flush toxins and promote a balanced inflammatory response.

12. Experiment and Be Creative:

- Experiment with different ingredients and recipes without fear. You can increase the sustainability and enjoyment of your anti-inflammatory diet by experimenting with different foods.

13. Mindful Eating:

- Eat mindfully by paying attention to hunger and fullness cues. Slow down and savor each bite, which can help you avoid overeating and make better food choices.

14. Consult a Dietitian:

- If you have specific health concerns or dietary restrictions, consider consulting a registered dietitian who can provide personalized guidance tailored to your needs.

15. Meal Prep and Batch Cooking:

   - Save time and make healthy eating more convenient by meal prepping and batch cooking. Prepare ingredients and meals in advance for the week.

By following these meal planning tips, you can make the transition to an anti-inflammatory diet smoother and more sustainable. It's a journey toward better health, and small, consistent changes in your eating habits can have a significant impact on reducing inflammation and improving your overall well-being.

CHAPTER 6: FREQUENTLY ASKED QUESTIONS

1. What is an anti-inflammatory diet?

   - An anti-inflammatory diet is a nutrition plan focused on reducing inflammation in the body by incorporating foods that have anti-inflammatory properties and avoiding those that can trigger inflammation.

2. What are the main principles of an anti-inflammatory diet?

   - The main principles include consuming more fruits and vegetables, healthy fats, whole grains, and lean proteins while limiting processed foods, sugars, and unhealthy fats.

3. Why is inflammation harmful to health?

   - Chronic inflammation is linked to various health issues, including heart disease, diabetes, autoimmune disorders, and certain cancers.

4. What foods should I avoid on an anti-inflammatory diet?

- Foods to limit or avoid include processed foods, sugary snacks and beverages, excessive saturated and trans fats, and refined grains.

5. What are the best anti-inflammatory foods to include in my diet?

- Anti-inflammatory foods include berries, fatty fish, leafy greens, turmeric, ginger, and olive oil, to name a few.

6. Can I drink alcohol on an anti-inflammatory diet?

- Alcohol should be consumed in moderation, as excessive alcohol can contribute to inflammation. Red wine in moderation may have some anti-inflammatory benefits.

7. How can I reduce inflammation through my diet?

- Reducing inflammation involves eating a balanced diet with a variety of anti-inflammatory foods, staying hydrated, and avoiding pro-inflammatory foods.

8. Are there specific diets that are considered anti-inflammatory, like the Mediterranean diet or the DASH diet?

  - Yes, diets like the Mediterranean diet and DASH diet are often considered anti-inflammatory due to their emphasis on whole foods, lean proteins, and healthy fats.

9. Can an anti-inflammatory diet help with weight loss?
- Yes, adopting an anti-inflammatory diet can support weight loss by promoting healthier food choices and reducing the risk of overeating.

10. Can an anti-inflammatory diet help with joint pain and arthritis?

  - Yes, an anti-inflammatory diet can potentially reduce joint pain and inflammation in conditions like arthritis.

11. Are there any supplements recommended for an anti-inflammatory diet?

  - While it's best to get nutrients from whole foods, some people may benefit from supplements like omega-3 fatty acids or curcumin (found in turmeric) to further reduce inflammation.

12. How long does it take to see the effects of an anti-inflammatory diet?   - It varies from person to person, but some individuals may start to feel improvements within a few weeks to a few months of adopting the diet.

13. Can an anti-inflammatory diet help with skin conditions like acne or psoriasis?

   - Yes, an anti-inflammatory diet can potentially improve skin conditions by reducing inflammation in the body.

14. Are there any restrictions on portion sizes in an anti-inflammatory diet?

   - Portion control is encouraged to avoid overeating, but there are no specific restrictions on portion sizes.

15. Is the anti-inflammatory diet suitable for vegetarians and vegans?

- Yes, the anti-inflammatory diet can be adapted for vegetarian and vegan lifestyles by incorporating plant-based sources of protein and healthy fats.

16. Can children follow an anti-inflammatory diet?

- An anti-inflammatory diet can be suitable for children, as it emphasizes nutrient-dense foods that are beneficial for growth and development.

17. Are there any potential side effects or drawbacks to the anti-inflammatory diet?

- While generally considered safe, some people may experience digestive changes as their bodies adjust to a diet high in fiber.

18. Can the anti-inflammatory diet be helpful for individuals with autoimmune diseases?

- It may help manage symptoms, but those with autoimmune diseases should consult with a healthcare professional before making significant dietary changes.

19. Are there any apps or tools to help with meal planning for an anti-inflammatory diet?

- Yes, there are several apps and online tools that can assist with meal planning and tracking nutrient intake.

20. How can I maintain an anti-inflammatory diet when dining out or traveling?

- Plan ahead, choose restaurants with healthier options, and make mindful menu selections. It's also a good idea to carry nutritious snacks when traveling.

CHAPTER 7: STAYING COMMITTED

Embarking on an anti-inflammatory diet is a profound commitment to your health and well-being. While the benefits are numerous, maintaining this dietary lifestyle can present challenges. Staying committed to an anti-inflammatory diet requires dedication, awareness, and a balanced approach. To assist you on your journey, consider the following advice:

1. Educate Yourself:

   - Knowledge is your best ally. Learn about the principles of the anti-inflammatory diet, its benefits, and the foods to include and avoid. Understanding the "why" behind your choices can help you stay committed.

2. Set Realistic Goals:

   - Establish achievable goals that align with your personal health and wellness objectives. Whether it's reducing joint pain, losing weight, or increasing energy levels, setting clear goals can keep you motivated.

3. Plan Your Meals:

   - Meal planning is essential. Plan your meals, create shopping lists, and prepare in advance. Having anti-inflammatory foods readily available makes it easier to stay on track.

4. Experiment with Recipes:

   - Variety is key to sustaining your commitment. Explore new recipes, ingredients, and cooking techniques. Discovering delicious, anti-inflammatory dishes can make your journey enjoyable.

5. Find Support:

   - Seek support from family, friends, or online communities who share your commitment to an anti-inflammatory lifestyle. Sharing experiences, recipes, and challenges can be motivating and reassuring.

6. Practice Mindful Eating:

- Pay attention to your body's hunger and fullness cues. Mindful eating can help you avoid overeating and make healthier choices.

7. Track Your Progress:

- Keep a journal to monitor how you feel, your energy levels, and any changes in your health. Celebrate your successes and use this feedback to adjust your approach.

8. Stay Hydrated:

- Drink plenty of water. Staying hydrated is vital for overall health, and it supports your body's natural processes, including inflammation control.

9. Be Patient and Forgiving:

- Understand that adapting to a new diet takes time. There may be moments when you deviate from your plan or face challenges. Be forgiving and refocus on your commitment.

10. Expert Advice: Take into account speaking with a licensed dietitian or other medical professional. They

can provide personalized guidance, tailor your diet to your specific needs, and address any concerns or questions.

11. Include Treats in Moderation:

   - It's okay to have occasional treats or indulge in your favorite foods, but do so in moderation. Allow yourself some flexibility while staying mindful of your overall dietary choices.

12. Positive Self-Talk:

   - Maintain a positive attitude. Encourage yourself and believe in your ability to stay committed. Self-compassion can help you navigate challenges.

13. Remember the Why:

   - Regularly remind yourself of the reasons you chose an anti-inflammatory diet. Whether it's better health, reduced pain, or enhanced vitality, keeping your motivations in mind can reinforce your commitment.

14. Seek Professional Guidance:

- If you encounter specific health concerns or dietary restrictions, consult with a healthcare professional or registered dietitian for personalized guidance and support.

Staying committed to an anti-inflammatory diet is a journey that may have its ups and downs, but it's a path toward greater well-being and vitality. By incorporating these tips and maintaining a balanced approach, you can not only enjoy the benefits of reduced inflammation but also develop a sustainable and healthful way of eating that serves you well in the long term.

www.ingramcontent.com/pod-product-compliance
Lightning Source LLC
Chambersburg PA
CBHW070841260726
48660CB00005B/2108